6-MINUTE ABS

Transform Your Core Fast

Get a Toned, Strong Core with Quick Workouts You Can Do Anywhere

SAM ERIC

DEDICATION

To my family, whose unwavering support and love have been my foundation,

To my friends, who have inspired and encouraged me every step of the way,

And to all the dreamers and doers, who strive for success and never give up,

This book is dedicated to you.

May it be a guide and a source of inspiration on your journey to achieving your dreams.

With heartfelt gratitude.

Abstract

Achieving a strong, toned core doesn't have to be time-consuming or complicated. *6-Minute Abs: Transform Your Core Fast* offers a practical, no-nonsense approach to strengthening your core in just six minutes a day. Designed for individuals with busy schedules, this guide breaks down the essentials of core training into manageable, effective routines that can be done anywhere—whether at home, in the gym, or even during a break at the office.

This book begins with foundational concepts, introducing readers to the anatomy of core muscles, the importance of core engagement, and proper breathing techniques to maximize workout efficiency. It explains how a strong core is essential not just for aesthetics but also for improved posture, enhanced athletic performance, and injury prevention.

The program is divided into progressive weekly plans, starting with basic exercises to build stability and proper form. As readers advance, they will encounter more dynamic and challenging routines designed to target all core muscle groups, including the rectus abdominis, obliques, transverse abdominis, and lower back muscles. Each routine is strategically crafted to deliver maximum results in minimal time, with options for modifications to suit all fitness levels.

Alongside the workout plans, *6-Minute Abs* emphasizes the role of consistency, proper nutrition, and mindfulness in achieving long-term results. It also includes troubleshooting tips for common mistakes, strategies to stay motivated, and insights into how core strength supports overall physical health.

With clear instructions, illustrative visuals, and motivational guidance, *6-Minute Abs: Transform Your Core Fast* empowers readers to take control of their fitness journey. Whether you're a beginner looking to start your fitness routine or an experienced athlete seeking to refine your core strength, this book delivers an efficient and sustainable path to a stronger, healthier core.

TABLE OF CONTENT

INTRODUCTION

Welcome to 6-Minute Abs: Transform Your Core Fast!, a powerful yet time-efficient guide to strengthening and toning your core. This book is designed to fit seamlessly into a busy lifestyle, making it possible for you to work on your core anywhere, anytime—even with just a few minutes to spare. Whether you're new to core workouts or an experienced fitness enthusiast, this program offers an adaptable, effective solution to build a strong, stable core that will benefit every area of your life.

Why a Strong Core Matters

A strong core is foundational to overall health, affecting posture, stability, mobility, and even breathing. The "core" includes not just the abdominal muscles but the entire network of muscles that support the spine and pelvis, including the lower back, obliques, hip flexors, and deep stabilizing muscles. Building a stronger core creates a ripple effect that benefits all movement patterns in daily life and physical activities. Here's why core strength is so essential:

- **Improved Posture**: A strong core helps maintain proper posture by aligning the spine and pelvis. Poor posture can lead to back, neck, and shoulder pain and create imbalances throughout the body. Core muscles work to support the spine and keep the body upright, preventing slouching and discomfort. Over time, enhanced posture from core strengthening can contribute to a healthier spine, better breathing, and a more confident stance.

- **Enhanced Stability and Balance**: Core strength provides a stable base for the body, allowing for controlled movement and balance. Whether you're reaching for something, twisting, or moving in multiple directions, the core muscles stabilize your movements, protecting against falls or strains. This is especially valuable in sports and physical activities, where dynamic movements require balance and coordination.
- **Injury Prevention**: Weak core muscles can lead to poor movement patterns, which increase the risk of injury, especially in the lower back. A strong core distributes the physical load across the body, reducing pressure on the spine, knees, and hips. This program helps create a balanced, stable core, which can prevent strains, sprains, and other injuries.

The 6-Minute Solution

In our busy lives, finding time to work out can be a challenge. The 6-Minute Abs program is designed to make core strengthening accessible, efficient, and effective. Each workout is only six minutes long, yet it's intense and targeted to achieve maximum results in minimal time.

The 6-minute approach is ideal for:

- **Busy Schedules**: Many people abandon fitness programs because they feel they don't have the time. This program is built for flexibility, allowing you to incorporate it whenever and wherever you have six minutes to spare.
- **Consistency and Long-Term Results**: Committing to a 6-minute workout is far more sustainable than longer routines. By maintaining a regular, brief workout, you create a habit that leads to long-term strength and toning.
- **Versatile Workout Options**: The exercises in this book require minimal or no equipment, making it easy to complete them at home, in the office, or even during travel.

This six-minute method also engages your core quickly and effectively, utilizing both endurance and strength-focused exercises. By cycling through various levels of difficulty, the program builds a strong core with routines that are accessible yet challenging.

Program Overview

The 6-Minute Abs program is designed for progression over six weeks, with each week focusing on different elements of core strength, stability, and conditioning. Here's what to expect from the program's structure:

- **Week 1: Building the Foundation** – This introductory week covers basic exercises that teach correct form, core engagement, and alignment. This foundation is essential to avoid injury and ensure you're effectively working the targeted muscles.
- **Week 2: Building Strength and Endurance** – Now that you have the basics, Week 2 introduces dynamic core exercises that build muscle strength and endurance. This phase increases intensity, helping you feel stronger and more capable.
- **Week 3: Targeting the Obliques and Lower Abs** – This week emphasizes the often-neglected obliques and lower abs, which are crucial for stability and creating a balanced, toned appearance.
- **Week 4: Advanced Core Conditioning** – For those looking for a challenge, Week 4 includes advanced exercises that require balance, control, and precision. These moves build endurance and stability, elevating your overall core strength.
- **Week 5: Cardio Core Blasts** – This week combines core exercises with cardio to increase calorie burn and improve cardiovascular endurance, providing a

more dynamic routine that helps sculpt the abs while supporting fat loss.

- **Week 6: Maintaining Core Health and Flexibility** – The final week includes core-strengthening moves combined with flexibility exercises to ensure you're keeping your core muscles strong, flexible, and balanced.

Each week introduces two to three different 6-minute routines, providing variety and keeping workouts fresh and engaging. You can follow along with the schedule or choose routines based on your goals and preferences.

Getting Started

Starting any fitness journey requires a plan. Here's how to set yourself up for success with the 6-Minute Abs program:

1. **Set Clear Goals**: Write down what you want to achieve with this program. Goals could be as specific as "improve posture" or "reduce lower back pain" or more general, like "feel stronger and more confident." Keeping goals clear will help you stay motivated.
2. **Create a Routine**: Determine when you'll complete your 6-minute workouts each day. Many people find it helpful to exercise first thing in the morning or during a midday

break to stay consistent. Set a timer or add it to your calendar as a non-negotiable task.

3. **Prepare Your Space**: Set up a designated workout area that's comfortable and free of distractions. If you're using equipment like a yoga mat or resistance bands, keep them nearby. Having a prepared space can make it easier to commit to the workout.

4. **Stay Consistent, Not Perfect**: The goal is to build a sustainable habit, so don't worry if you miss a day. Focus on showing up consistently, and your core will get stronger over time. Progress is gradual, and the key is to stay committed.

5. **Track Your Progress**: Use a notebook, journal, or fitness app to record your workouts, note any improvements, and reflect on how you feel after each session. Tracking your progress will allow you to see results, stay motivated, and adjust your goals as you go.

6. **Focus on Quality Over Quantity**: With each session being only six minutes, it's crucial to maintain proper form and engage the core muscles effectively. Taking a moment to focus on your breathing, alignment, and core engagement before each exercise will maximize your results.

With this program, you're setting out on a fast, efficient, and empowering journey to transform your core. Six minutes a day is all it takes to strengthen, stabilize, and sculpt, helping you create the foundation for a healthier, more resilient body. Let's get started and make every second count!

Week 1: Building the Foundation

Goal: Establish basic core activation, stability, and form.

Chapter 1: Core Basics – Understanding Your Core Muscles

In this first chapter, you'll gain a foundational understanding of your core anatomy and learn key techniques for engaging your core muscles effectively. These basics will help you build stability, improve your form, and set the stage for a safe, productive workout experience throughout this program.

Overview of Core Muscles

The core is more than just the "abs"—it's a complex network of muscles that work together to support posture, balance, and stability. Each muscle plays a unique role:

- **Rectus Abdominis**: Often referred to as the "six-pack," this is the long, flat muscle on the front of the abdomen. It assists in bending the spine forward and is essential for core stability.
- **Transverse Abdominis**: Located beneath the rectus abdominis, this is the

deepest abdominal muscle. Often called the "corset muscle," it wraps around the spine for support and is crucial for core stability and lower back health.

- **Obliques**: These muscles are on each side of the abdomen. There are two types—external and internal obliques. They assist in twisting and bending movements and play an important role in stabilizing the spine during side-to-side movements.
- **Lower Back (Erector Spinae and Multifidus)**: While often overlooked, the lower back muscles are critical to a balanced core. They run along the spine and help in extending and stabilizing the back. Strengthening these muscles helps prevent back injuries and promotes good posture.

A balanced approach to core strengthening means working all these muscles harmoniously. Weakness in any part of the core can lead to imbalances, which can cause pain or increase the risk of injury. By understanding each muscle's function, you'll be better prepared to focus on activation and engagement, maximizing results while minimizing strain.

Engagement Techniques

Knowing how to engage your core is key to achieving effective, safe results. Many people mistakenly rely on their upper body or legs rather than fully activating their core. Here are foundational techniques for proper engagement:

1. **Draw-In Maneuver**: Imagine pulling your belly button in toward your spine. This action engages the transverse abdominis, stabilizing the entire core area. Practice this in a standing or seated position before progressing to exercises.
2. **Pelvic Tilt**: This move helps to activate the lower abdominals. While lying on your back with knees bent, press your lower back into the ground, tilting your pelvis slightly upward. This tilt can be felt in exercises like bridges and leg raises, where core stability is crucial.
3. **Bracing**: Think of tightening your core as if you're about to be lightly punched in the stomach. You should feel all your core muscles tighten, not just the abs. This engagement technique helps protect the spine during exercises.
4. **Mindful Engagement**: Focus on which muscles you're activating as you move. During each exercise, bring awareness to the muscles working. This not only improves form but also builds a stronger mind-body connection, making your workouts more effective.

Remember, effective core work is about precision, not speed. Start with these techniques and integrate them into each movement for optimal muscle engagement.

The Importance of Breathing

Breathing correctly enhances core engagement, endurance, and overall performance. Coordinated breathing with core engagement also helps regulate oxygen flow, making exercises safer and more effective. Here's how to use breathing to your advantage in core workouts:

1. **Diaphragmatic Breathing**: Also known as belly breathing, this technique promotes core activation by engaging the diaphragm. Inhale deeply through the nose, expanding the belly as you fill the diaphragm with air. Exhale fully through the mouth, drawing the belly button toward the spine. Practicing this breathing style before workouts will build endurance and prepare your core for activation.
2. **Inhale to Prepare, Exhale to Engage**: For most core exercises, it's best to inhale before starting the movement and exhale during the effort phase. For example, when performing a crunch, inhale as you lower, then exhale as you lift. This not only improves control but also ensures a deep core engagement, stabilizing your movements.

3. **Breath Control for Endurance**: Holding your breath during a workout can limit oxygen flow and create unnecessary tension. Maintaining steady, rhythmic breathing helps regulate heart rate and enhances endurance, allowing you to complete exercises without straining.
4. **Mindful Exhalation for Core Activation**: Exhaling sharply while performing an intense part of an exercise, like contracting at the top of a crunch, helps deepen core engagement. This exhalation technique activates the transverse abdominis and rectus abdominis, making your workout more effective.

Proper breathing can make a noticeable difference in the quality of each workout, reducing fatigue and supporting the core from the inside out.

By understanding core anatomy, engagement techniques, and the power of breath, you're building a strong foundation for safe and effective workouts. These fundamentals will carry you through the program, helping you get the most out of every 6-minute session as you work toward a stronger, more resilient core.

Chapter 2: Foundational Exercises for Beginners

This chapter introduces you to beginner-friendly core exercises, each designed to build a solid foundation in form, stability, and endurance. With detailed step-by-step breakdowns, form and alignment tips, and 6-minute routines, you'll gain confidence in basic moves that form the backbone of an effective core workout.

Exercise Breakdown: Step-by-Step Guides

Each of the following exercises is crafted to activate and strengthen different parts of your core, promoting muscle balance and coordination. Here's how to perform each exercise with correct form:

1. **Plank**

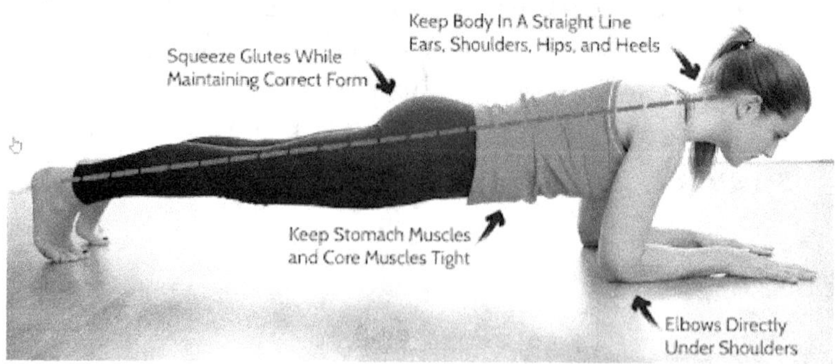

- **Purpose**: Strengthens the entire core, focusing on stability.
- **Steps**:
    1. Start on all fours, aligning shoulders directly over wrists and knees under hips.
    2. Extend legs back, lifting knees off the floor and keeping your body in a straight line from head to heels.
    3. Engage your core by pulling the belly button toward the spine, squeeze glutes, and press hands firmly into the floor.
    4. Hold this position for 10–30 seconds, gradually increasing time as you build strength.
- **Muscles Targeted**: Rectus abdominis, transverse abdominis, shoulders, glutes.

2. **Modified Crunch**

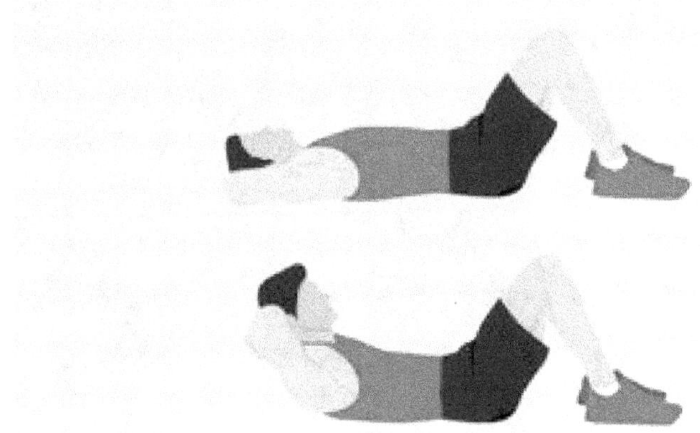

- **Purpose**: Activates the upper and lower abs in a controlled, low-impact movement.
- **Steps**:
    1. Lie on your back with knees bent and feet flat on the floor, hip-width apart.
    2. Place your hands behind your head for support, with elbows pointing outward.
    3. Inhale, then exhale as you lift your head, neck, and shoulders slightly off the ground, keeping the lower back pressed into the floor.
    4. Hold briefly at the top, engaging your abs, then inhale as you lower back down slowly.
- **Muscles Targeted**: Rectus abdominis, transverse abdominis.

3. **Dead Bug**

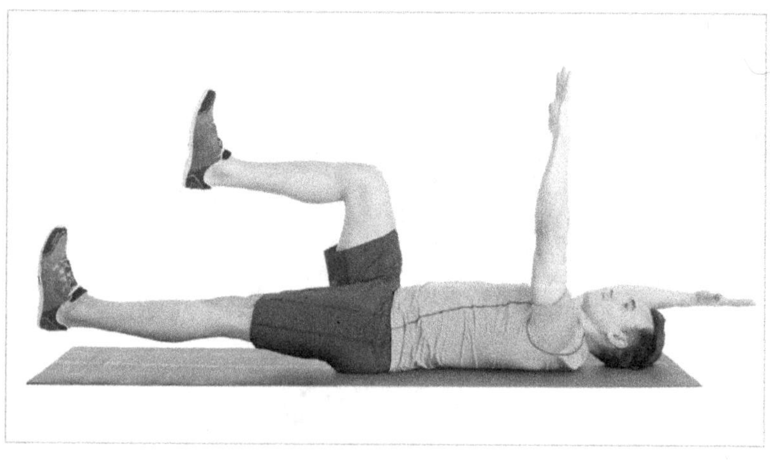

- o **Purpose**: Strengthens deep core muscles and improves coordination.
- o **Steps**:
    1. Lie on your back with arms extended toward the ceiling and knees bent at a 90-degree angle.
    2. Engage your core, keeping your lower back pressed against the floor.
    3. Slowly lower your right arm and left leg toward the floor without arching the back.
    4. Return to the starting position and switch sides, lowering the left arm and right leg.
- o **Muscles Targeted**: Transverse abdominis, rectus abdominis, obliques.

These foundational exercises emphasize form and steady engagement, providing a low-impact way to start building core strength.

Form and Alignment Tips

Proper form and alignment are essential to avoiding injury and maximizing results. Here are key tips for each of the exercises:

- **Plank**: Keep a straight line from head to heels without letting hips sag or rise.

Imagine pulling your belly button up toward your spine to engage your core effectively.

- **Modified Crunch**: Avoid pulling on the neck with your hands, which can strain the neck muscles. Instead, use your core muscles to lift your torso, keeping your chin slightly tucked.
- **Dead Bug**: Maintain a flat lower back against the floor throughout the movement. If the back arches, reduce the range of motion until core strength improves.

Focusing on these form tips allows you to target your muscles properly while avoiding common mistakes.

6-Minute Workout Routines

These two routines introduce you to core-focused movements in short, manageable sessions. Practice them on alternate days to build strength and confidence as you start your journey.

Routine 1: Core Activation and Stability

1. **Plank** – 30 seconds
2. **Modified Crunch** – 12 reps
3. **Dead Bug** – 10 reps per side

Repeat this circuit twice, resting for 30 seconds between rounds.

Routine 2: Endurance and Control

1. **Modified Crunch** – 15 reps
2. **Dead Bug** – 10 reps per side
3. **Plank** – 20 seconds, rest for 10 seconds, then 20 more seconds

Repeat this circuit twice, resting for 30 seconds between rounds.

These routines are designed to give you a well-rounded introduction to core work, focusing on activating the muscles and practicing correct form and breathing. The short time commitment and steady approach help you master the basics before moving on to more challenging exercises. Over time, you'll build strength, endurance, and confidence in your core workouts.

Week 2: Building Strength and Endurance

Goal: Increase core strength and endurance through more dynamic exercises.

Chapter 3: Increasing Intensity Safely

This chapter focuses on safely advancing your core workouts. As you build strength and confidence in your foundational exercises, gradual progression is key to continued improvement. Here, you'll learn essential principles for safely increasing intensity, along with practical modifications to adapt exercises to your evolving abilities.

Progression Principles: How to Advance Exercises Safely and Effectively

As you progress, making gradual changes to exercise difficulty, duration, or resistance can help you avoid plateaus while minimizing the risk of injury. Here are key principles for progressing your core workouts effectively:

1. **Increase Reps or Hold Time Gradually**

- o Adding extra repetitions or holding each pose slightly longer is a safe way to increase intensity without drastically changing the movement. For example, if you've been holding a plank for 20 seconds, try increasing to 30 seconds, then to 45 as you feel stronger.
- o **Example**: Start with 10 reps of the Dead Bug, then increase by 2 reps each week as your stability improves.

2. **Incorporate Variations**
- o Introducing small variations to your exercises targets different muscle fibers and improves overall core endurance and strength. For instance, adding a knee tap to the plank or a twist to the crunch can intensify the workout without requiring new equipment.
- o **Example**: Try a Side Plank for 10–20 seconds on each side to engage the obliques and add lateral core stability.

3. **Increase Range of Motion**
- o For exercises like crunches or leg lifts, extending the range of motion helps recruit more muscle fibers. Moving through a larger range, however, requires more control, so only progress when you feel stable and maintain form.
- o **Example**: In a crunch, gradually lift the torso higher or extend legs lower

in the Dead Bug for a greater range of movement.

4. **Add Controlled Movements**
   - Combining movements, like adding a knee-to-elbow tap in a plank or a slight leg lift in a crunch, increases complexity and requires more coordination. Ensure you can perform each individual movement confidently before combining them.
   - **Example**: For the Plank, add a shoulder tap every few seconds to engage more muscles while maintaining stability.

Remember, progression is about gradual, steady improvement. Listen to your body, and don't rush to the next level until you feel strong and stable with the current intensity.

Intensity Modifications: Adjusting Exercises for Different Levels and Abilities

Each body responds differently to exercise, so it's essential to modify intensity based on personal ability, ensuring that the exercises remain challenging but safe. Here are ways to adjust the intensity of common core exercises:

1. **Modifications for Plank**

- o **Beginner**: Start on your knees rather than toes, reducing the load on your core and upper body.
- o **Intermediate**: Try the standard plank on your toes, aiming to maintain proper alignment for 20–30 seconds.
- o **Advanced**: Increase the difficulty by lifting one leg slightly off the ground or adding shoulder taps for additional balance and core control.

2. **Modifications for Crunch**
- o **Beginner**: Start with a very shallow crunch, lifting only the shoulders and upper back off the mat, focusing on controlled movement.
- o **Intermediate**: Lift higher, engaging the full upper body while keeping the lower back pressed into the mat.
- o **Advanced**: Add a twist at the top, aiming one elbow toward the opposite knee for an oblique crunch, or perform a "bicycle crunch" to engage multiple core muscles in a single movement.

3. **Modifications for Dead Bug**
- o **Beginner**: Perform the exercise with just the arms or legs moving, not both at once, to develop stability.
- o **Intermediate**: Alternate lowering opposite arm and leg while keeping the core engaged, focusing on slow, controlled movements.

- o **Advanced**: Lower the arm and leg closer to the floor while maintaining a stable, flat back, which intensifies the effort required from the transverse abdominis.

4. **Modifications for Side Plank**
   - o **Beginner**: Keep the bottom knee on the ground, forming a supported side plank that provides more stability.
   - o **Intermediate**: Straighten both legs, stacking feet one over the other and supporting yourself on one arm.
   - o **Advanced**: Add a leg lift with the top leg or rotate the torso slightly toward the ground for a challenging dynamic side plank.

These adjustments and modifications allow you to customize your workout based on your fitness level, ensuring that each session remains challenging and productive. Progressing safely ensures that you're building a core that is not only strong but balanced and resilient, able to support the body through a wide range of movements and physical demands.

Chapter 4: Dynamic Core Exercises

In Chapter 4, we'll dive into intermediate-level core exercises that bring more dynamic movement into your workout. This progression introduces you to exercises that build strength, coordination, and endurance by incorporating controlled motion. Through compound exercises, you'll learn how to target multiple muscles efficiently, creating a strong and stable core in just a few minutes a day.

Introduction to Intermediate Moves

The following exercises require slightly more coordination and endurance than beginner moves, making them ideal for intermediate-level training. Each of these exercises engages multiple core muscles, helping to strengthen the abs, obliques, and back while challenging your stability and control.

1. **Bicycle Crunch**
     - **Purpose**: Engages both the rectus abdominis and obliques through twisting and leg movement.
     - **Steps**:
          1. Lie on your back with knees bent and hands behind your head.
          2. Lift your head, neck, and shoulders off the mat, bringing

your right elbow toward your left knee as you extend your right leg.

3. Switch sides, bringing your left elbow to your right knee as you extend your left leg.

4. Continue alternating in a smooth, controlled motion, as if pedaling a bicycle.

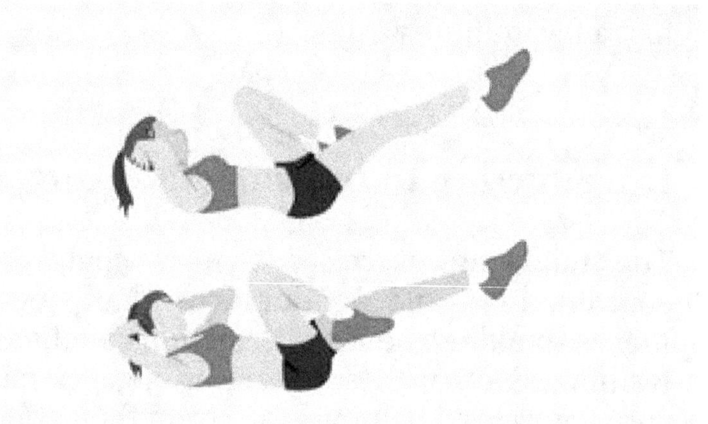

- **Tip**: Move slowly to maximize muscle engagement, keeping your lower back pressed into the mat.

2. **Russian Twist**
   - **Purpose**: Targets the obliques, improving rotational strength and stability.
   - **Steps**:
     1. Sit on the floor with knees bent and feet flat.

2. Lean back slightly, keeping your spine straight and core engaged.
3. Hold your hands together at your chest, or hold a small weight if desired.
4. Rotate your torso to the right, bringing your hands toward the floor beside you, then return to the center and twist to the left.

- **Tip**: Engage your core and avoid rounding the back. For added difficulty, lift your feet off the floor to balance on your sit bones.

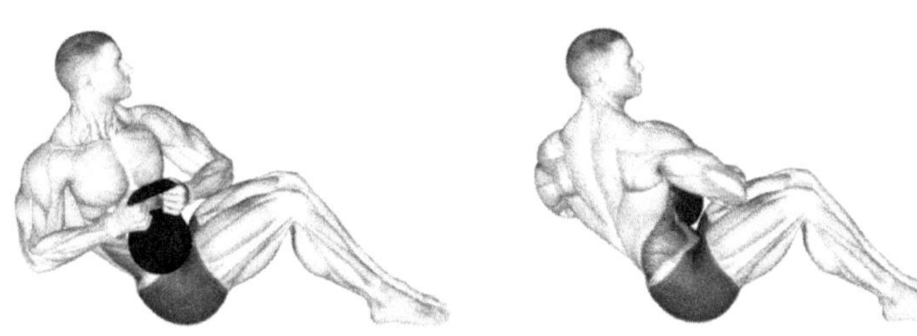

3. **Mountain Climbers**
   - **Purpose**: Engages the entire core while building cardiovascular endurance and lower body strength.
   - **Steps**:
     1. Start in a high plank position, with hands under shoulders and body in a straight line.
     2. Drive your right knee toward your chest, then quickly switch

legs, bringing your left knee in as you extend the right leg back.

3. Continue alternating knees at a steady pace, keeping the core tight and avoiding a sagging back.

- **Tip**: Keep your hips level, focusing on core stability over speed.

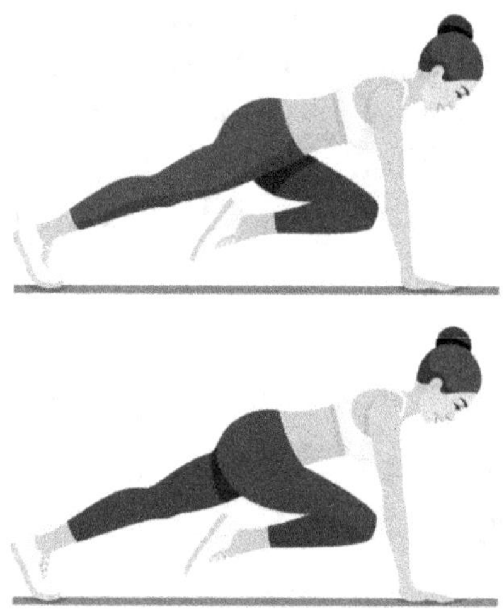

These dynamic exercises are excellent for challenging the body's stability while increasing heart rate, making them ideal for a short, effective workout.

Combining Movements for Efficiency

Compound movements are excellent for maximizing results in a short time. By combining exercises, you can target multiple muscle groups at once, enhancing core strength and promoting balance throughout the body. Here's how each of these dynamic moves promotes efficiency:

- **Bicycle Crunch**: Combines twisting and leg motion, targeting both the upper and lower abs along with the obliques.
- **Russian Twist**: Adds rotational movement, engaging the entire core, especially the obliques, while also requiring lower back stability.
- **Mountain Climbers**: Integrates core activation with cardiovascular engagement, increasing core endurance while also working hip flexors and shoulders.

Adding these exercises into your routine makes each minute count, giving you the most out of every workout session.

6-Minute Workout Routines

These two intermediate routines combine dynamic movements, designed to challenge your strength, coordination, and endurance in a brief, intense workout.

Routine 1: Core Burn and Twist

1. **Bicycle Crunch** – 30 seconds
2. **Russian Twist** – 30 seconds
3. **Mountain Climbers** – 30 seconds

Rest for 15 seconds and repeat the circuit twice, adjusting rest as needed.

Routine 2: Full-Core Engagement

1. **Mountain Climbers** – 30 seconds
2. **Bicycle Crunch** – 30 seconds
3. **Russian Twist** – 30 seconds

Rest for 15 seconds and repeat the circuit twice.

These routines are short but intense, focusing on dynamic movements that boost endurance and build a stable core. Incorporating these exercises into your routine will increase overall strength while helping you develop a core that can handle both static and dynamic demands. Remember, form is key; keep movements controlled to ensure maximum benefit and safety.

Week 3: Targeting the Obliques and Lower Abs

Goal: Emphasize lower abdominal and oblique activation for balanced core development.

Chapter 5: The Role of Obliques and Lower Abs in Core Stability

In Chapter 5, we focus on the obliques and lower abdominal muscles, often overlooked but essential for core stability. These muscles support functional movement, posture, and balance while providing strength and control to rotational and side-bending movements. Developing these muscles properly enhances overall core stability, which is crucial for injury prevention and daily activities.

Understanding the Muscles: How Obliques and Lower Abs Contribute to a Balanced and Stable Core

The core consists of multiple muscle groups working in harmony, and the obliques and lower abs play a vital role in this integrated system:

1. **Obliques**
   - The obliques are divided into the **internal** and **external obliques**,

located along the sides of the abdomen. They allow the torso to rotate, twist, and bend to the side and stabilize the body during these movements.

- **External Obliques**: These are the outermost layer and are activated during movements that involve trunk rotation or lateral flexion (side bending).
- **Internal Obliques**: Located beneath the external obliques, these muscles work synergistically with them and aid in stabilizing the spine during twisting and bending.
- **Importance for Core Stability**: The obliques help balance the upper body over the pelvis and prevent unwanted rotation or sway. They're especially crucial in athletic activities or movements requiring power, such as lifting, throwing, or sprinting.

2. **Lower Abdominals**
   - The **lower abs** are primarily the lower portion of the **rectus abdominis** and part of the **transverse abdominis**. They stabilize the pelvis and spine, especially in lower-body movements and activities that challenge balance.
   - **Rectus Abdominis (Lower Portion)**: Commonly associated with "six-pack" muscles, the lower part is responsible for flexing the

lumbar spine, particularly during leg lifts or knee tucks.

- o **Transverse Abdominis (TVA)**: This deep layer wraps around the abdomen and acts like a corset, pulling the belly inward and providing stability for the spine and pelvis. Engaging the TVA is crucial for lower ab engagement and core stability.
- o **Importance for Core Stability**: Lower abs help prevent excessive arching of the lower back and maintain spinal alignment. They play a key role in stabilizing the lower body and core during movement and exercise, reducing strain on the lower back.

Common Mistakes: Tips to Avoid When Targeting the Obliques and Lower Abs

To effectively strengthen the obliques and lower abs, form and engagement are critical. Many people unknowingly make mistakes that reduce the efficacy of exercises or even increase injury risk. Here's what to watch out for:

1. **Over-Rotating in Oblique Exercises**
   - o **Mistake**: Twisting too far in exercises like Bicycle Crunch or Russian Twist, which can strain the

lower back and diminish core engagement.

- o **Tip**: Focus on controlled, intentional movement, keeping the range of motion within a comfortable range. Aim for rotation that feels like it's coming from the core, not the shoulders.

2. **Using Momentum in Lower Ab Exercises**
   - o **Mistake**: Swinging the legs or using momentum during exercises like Leg Raises or Reverse Crunch, which can strain the lower back.
   - o **Tip**: Move slowly and with control. Keep the lower back pressed into the mat to protect the spine and maximize lower ab engagement. Lower your legs as far as you can without your back lifting off the mat.

3. **Failing to Engage the Transverse Abdominis**
   - o **Mistake**: Not engaging the deep core muscles, particularly the TVA, during exercises that target the lower abs. This can lead to an arched lower back and less core stability.
   - o **Tip**: Before each movement, pull the navel inward toward the spine, as if you're tightening a belt around your waist. This engages the TVA and stabilizes the spine.

4. **Straining the Neck in Oblique Crunches**

- o **Mistake**: Pulling on the neck during twisting movements, which can lead to discomfort and misalignment.
  - o **Tip**: Keep the head aligned with the spine and let the core initiate the movement. Lightly place your hands behind your head without pulling forward.
5. **Neglecting Breath Control**
  - o **Mistake**: Holding your breath during challenging moves, which reduces oxygen flow and leads to faster fatigue.
  - o **Tip**: Exhale during the exertion phase of the movement (e.g., twisting up in a Bicycle Crunch or lifting legs in a Leg Raise) and inhale during the release. Proper breathing will increase endurance and help engage the core muscles.

By understanding the role of the obliques and lower abs and avoiding common mistakes, you can engage these muscles effectively and safely, creating a strong, stable, and balanced core. With these fundamentals in mind, you'll be able to execute exercises with optimal form, maximizing the benefits and strengthening your core to support your body in everyday movements and fitness pursuits.

Chapter 6: Lower Ab and Oblique Exercises

In Chapter 6, we focus on specific exercises that target the obliques and lower abs, essential areas for core stability, balance, and strength. Strengthening these muscles improves your ability to stabilize the spine and pelvis, enhances your posture, and supports more effective movement in daily activities. Each exercise in this chapter is designed to engage the lower abdominal muscles and obliques with precision, helping you build a stable core with simple yet effective movements.

Specific Exercises: Focused Moves for Obliques and Lower Abs

1. Side Plank

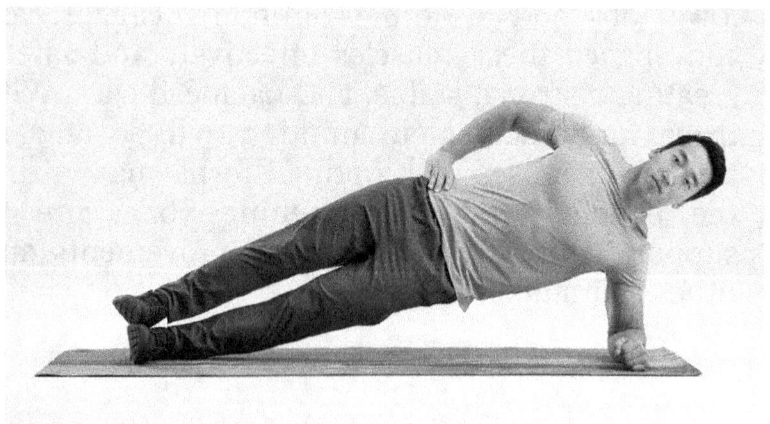

- Purpose: Strengthens the obliques,
  improves balance, and enhances
  stability.
- **Steps**:
    1. Start by lying on your side,
       with your elbow directly under
       your shoulder and legs stacked.
    2. Engage your core and lift your
       hips off the floor, creating a
       straight line from head to feet.
    3. Hold for 15–30 seconds,
       maintaining a stable torso and
       avoiding sagging at the hips.
    4. Repeat on the opposite side.
- **Modification**: Drop the bottom
  knee to the floor for additional
  support, making it easier to hold the
  position while focusing on oblique
  engagement.
- **Tip**: Keep your body aligned and
  avoid collapsing the shoulder by
  pushing the supporting arm down
  into the floor.

2. **Leg Raises**
   - **Purpose**: Targets the lower abs,
     promoting pelvic stability and core
     strength.
   - **Steps**:
       1. Lie on your back with your legs
          extended and arms by your
          sides.
       2. Slowly lift both legs toward the
          ceiling while keeping them

straight and engaging your lower abs.

3. Lower your legs back down in a controlled motion, stopping just before they touch the floor to maintain tension in the core.

- o **Modification**: Bend your knees slightly for a gentler variation, or place your hands under your lower back for extra support.
- o **Tip**: Avoid arching the lower back; keep it pressed gently into the mat by tightening your core.

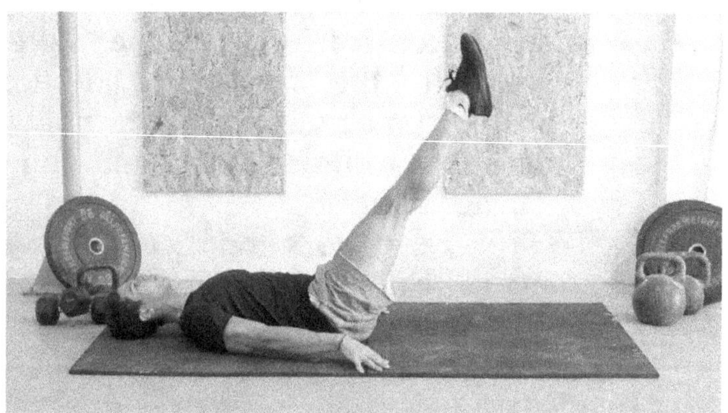

3. **Heel Taps**
    - o **Purpose**: Strengthens the lower abs with minimal strain on the neck and back.
    - o **Steps**:
        1. Lie on your back with your knees bent at 90 degrees and legs lifted so your shins are parallel to the floor.

2. Engage your core, then slowly lower one heel toward the floor while keeping the other leg in place.
   3. Tap the floor lightly with your heel, then bring the leg back to the starting position and switch sides.
   - **Modification**: Perform this movement with both feet on the floor, lifting one leg at a time if it's challenging to keep the back flat.
   - **Tip**: Move slowly to avoid using momentum, allowing the lower abs to stay engaged throughout the motion.

These exercises provide targeted engagement for the obliques and lower abs, creating a strong foundation for core stability and balanced strength.

6-Minute Workout Routines

Below are two efficient 6-minute routines designed to build strength in the obliques and lower abs. Each workout combines the exercises above into a time-saving routine that can be done anywhere with no equipment.

Routine 1: Oblique Power

1. **Side Plank (Right Side)** – 30 seconds
2. **Side Plank (Left Side)** – 30 seconds
3. **Heel Taps** – 30 seconds
4. **Side Plank (Right Side)** – 30 seconds
5. **Side Plank (Left Side)** – 30 seconds
6. **Heel Taps** – 30 seconds

Repeat for one circuit. Rest as needed between exercises to maintain form.

Routine 2: Lower Ab Challenge

1. **Leg Raises** – 30 seconds
2. **Heel Taps** – 30 seconds
3. **Side Plank (Right Side)** – 30 seconds
4. **Leg Raises** – 30 seconds
5. **Heel Taps** – 30 seconds
6. **Side Plank (Left Side)** – 30 seconds

Complete one circuit, focusing on controlled, mindful movement.

These routines can be incorporated into your weekly workouts or used as standalone sessions to build a strong foundation in your core. By practicing these moves regularly, you'll gain greater strength, balance, and control over your core muscles, setting the stage for advanced stability and overall fitness. Remember to prioritize form over speed, as slow and intentional movements yield the best results for targeting the obliques and lower abs.

Week 4: Advanced Core Conditioning

Goal: Incorporate advanced exercises that challenge stability, control, and strength for total core transformation.

Chapter 7: Stability and Control – Key Elements of Core Conditioning

In Chapter 7, we focus on the importance of stability and control in core conditioning. Stability and control are the foundation for a balanced, injury-resistant body, enhancing the ability to perform everyday tasks and supporting athletic performance. By learning to activate and control deep stabilizing muscles, you'll build core strength that translates into better posture, improved coordination, and greater efficiency in movement.

The Importance of Stability in Functional Fitness

How Improved Control Translates to Daily Activities and Athletic Performance

1. **Enhanced Movement Efficiency**
   Stability is crucial in supporting functional fitness, which refers to strength, flexibility, and endurance that assist in daily tasks and

physical activities. A stable core allows the body to move more efficiently, whether you're lifting, bending, or twisting. By stabilizing your torso, the core minimizes unnecessary movement, enabling more precise and effective actions in both simple tasks like bending down and more complex activities like running or jumping.

2. **Injury Prevention**
   Core stability helps protect the spine and pelvis by providing a stable base from which the arms and legs can operate safely. Poor core stability can lead to compensations in other muscles, which increases the risk of injuries, especially in the lower back and hips. By focusing on stability and control exercises, you strengthen the muscles that support the spine and reduce the likelihood of strains, sprains, and overuse injuries.

3. **Support for Athletic Performance**
   Athletes in any sport rely on core stability for peak performance. In sports that involve running, jumping, or rotational movements (like tennis or golf), stability provides a foundation for explosive movements and helps athletes control their motion with precision. For example, a soccer player can maintain stability through the core while kicking or pivoting, leading to improved accuracy, power, and agility. Developing core control allows you to handle quick changes in direction, high-

intensity movements, and repetitive motions without risking form breakdown.

Body Awareness and Control

How to Engage Deep Stabilizing Muscles for Improved Balance and Coordination

1. **Understanding the Role of Deep Core Muscles**
   The deep core muscles—including the transverse abdominis, multifidus, and pelvic floor—are often less visible but play a vital role in stabilization. These muscles act as a natural corset for the spine, providing support from within, which allows the outer muscles (like the rectus abdominis and obliques) to perform more dynamic movements. Learning to engage these stabilizers is key to developing a strong core foundation.

2. **Building Body Awareness for Better Engagement**
   Body awareness is the ability to sense where your body is in space and how it moves. Developing awareness in your core muscles is essential for engaging the right muscles at the right times. Breathing techniques can assist in this process, as exhaling during exertion can activate the transverse abdominis, helping you achieve a braced, stable position. Practicing slower,

controlled movements like planks or bird-dog variations also encourages you to "feel" the muscles working, improving your connection to the core.

3. **Control and Coordination in Motion** Stability in motion—such as maintaining a strong core during a twisting movement—relies on coordination. Exercises that involve small, controlled shifts in weight, like single-leg balance exercises or dynamic planks, teach the core muscles to respond to change while maintaining control. These exercises also build neuromuscular coordination, helping you stay stable even when facing unexpected movements or changes in direction.

Key Exercises for Stability and Control

This chapter includes exercises specifically designed to enhance stability, body awareness, and control through mindful engagement of the deep core muscles:

1. **Bird-Dog**
   - **Purpose**: Engages the lower back and core while promoting balance.
   - **Execution**:
     1. Start on your hands and knees, keeping your spine neutral.

2. Extend one arm forward while extending the opposite leg straight back.
3. Hold for a moment, maintaining stability, then return to the starting position and switch sides.

- o **Tip**: Keep your core engaged to prevent arching the lower back.

2. **Dead Bug**
   - o **Purpose**: Strengthens the deep core muscles while teaching control over limb movements.
   - o **Execution**:
     1. Lie on your back with your arms extended above and legs in a tabletop position.
     2. Slowly lower one arm and the opposite leg toward the floor while keeping the lower back flat.
     3. Return to the starting position and repeat with the other side.
   - o **Tip**: Move slowly to maintain core engagement without straining the lower back.

3. **Side Plank with Knee Tuck**
   - o **Purpose**: Targets the obliques while challenging balance and stability.
   - o **Execution**:
     1. Begin in a side plank with your elbow under your shoulder and legs stacked.

2. Draw the top knee toward your chest, then return it to the starting position.
3. Repeat for several reps, then switch sides.

- o **Tip**: Focus on keeping your hips lifted to maintain alignment.

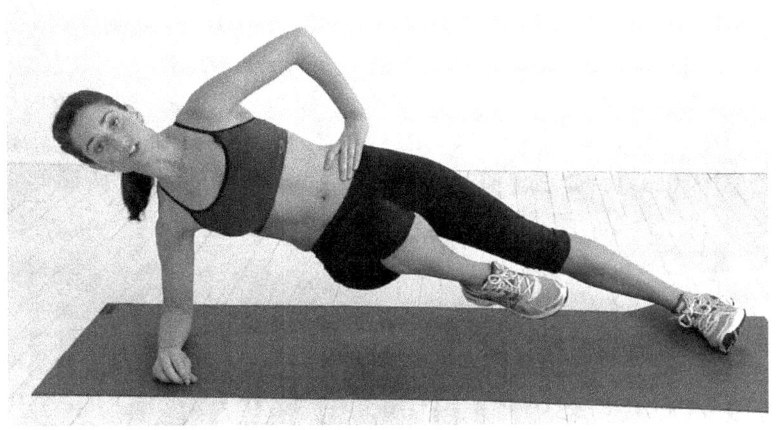

By practicing these stability and control exercises, you'll build a core that is both resilient and adaptable, supporting you in a range of physical activities. This foundation allows you to approach more challenging movements with confidence, knowing your core can maintain balance, coordination, and alignment under varying conditions. The resulting strength and stability will benefit not only your workouts but also everyday activities, fostering long-term core health and performance.

Chapter 8: Advanced Core Exercises

In Chapter 8, we explore advanced core exercises that challenge stability, endurance, and control, elevating your core strength to a higher level. This chapter introduces exercises that engage multiple muscle groups through dynamic and complex movements, building resilience and coordination in the core. These advanced routines are crafted to push your limits safely, providing effective workouts for those who have mastered foundational exercises and are ready for more intensity.

Advanced Movements

Exercises like Plank Variations, Jackknife, and V-Ups

1. Plank Variations

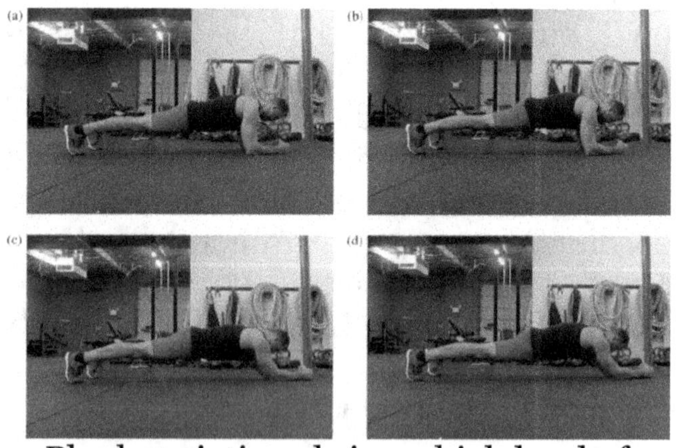

Plank variations bring a high level of

engagement across the core and target both stability and strength. Here are some advanced options:

- **Plank to Pike**:
    - **Purpose**: Engages the upper and lower core, along with the shoulders.
    - **Execution**: Start in a high plank position. Draw your hips upward toward the ceiling into a pike position, keeping your legs straight. Lower back down to plank and repeat.
    - **Tip**: Move slowly to control the descent, avoiding any strain on the lower back.
- **Shoulder Tap Plank**:
    - **Purpose**: Enhances stability and balance, working the obliques and deeper stabilizers.
    - **Execution**: In a high plank, lift one hand to tap the opposite shoulder while keeping hips steady. Alternate sides.
    - **Tip**: Avoid rocking the hips; focus on core control.

2. **Jackknife**
The jackknife exercise engages the entire core, especially targeting the lower abs through an intense lifting motion.

- o **Purpose**: Builds strength in the upper and lower core, with a focus on controlled movements.
- o **Execution**: Lie on your back with arms extended overhead. Simultaneously lift your legs and arms, reaching toward the toes at the top. Lower down slowly and repeat.
- o **Tip**: Keep your movements slow to control engagement and avoid using momentum.

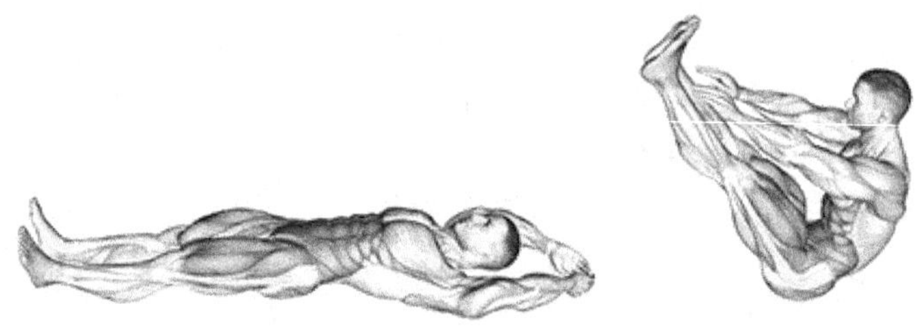

3. **V-Ups**

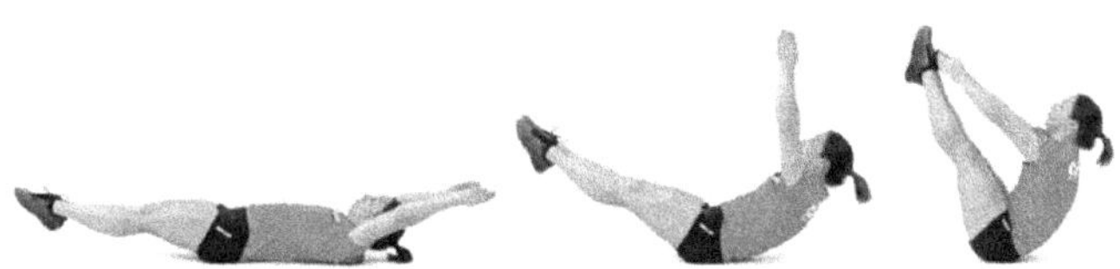

V-Ups challenge both core strength and flexibility, requiring controlled movement through the entire torso.

- o **Purpose**: Activates the rectus abdominis, obliques, and hip flexors, building explosive core power.
- o **Execution**: Begin lying flat on your back with arms extended overhead and legs straight. Simultaneously lift your legs and torso, reaching your hands toward your toes to form a "V" shape. Lower back down and repeat.
- o **Tip**: Keep your lower back engaged and avoid arching as you lower down.

Balance and Control Moves

Balancing Exercises to Engage Deeper Stabilizers

1. **Single-Leg Plank**

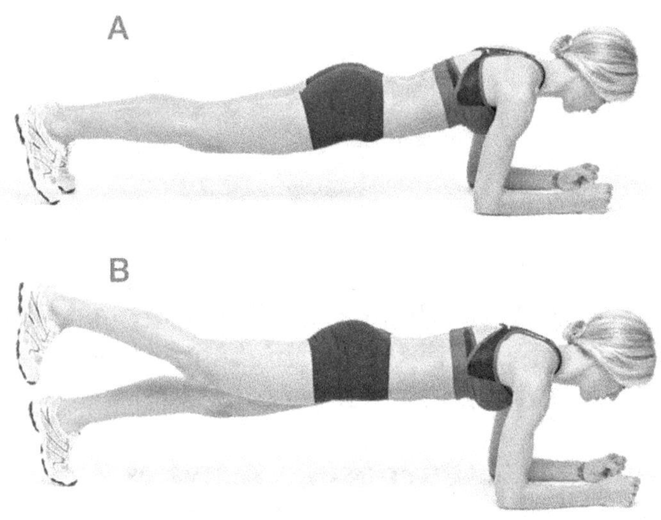

By removing one point of stability, this exercise engages the obliques and deep core stabilizers, improving balance and coordination.

- **Execution**: Start in a high plank position. Lift one leg slightly off the ground and hold, maintaining a steady core. Switch legs after several breaths.
- **Tip**: Keep your hips level to prevent shifting or tilting.

2. **Side Plank with Leg Lift**

This variation of the side plank engages the

obliques and hip muscles while improving balance.

- o **Execution**: Begin in a side plank with your bottom elbow directly below your shoulder. Lift your top leg toward the ceiling while keeping your body aligned. Hold for a moment, then return to the starting position.
- o **Tip**: Engage the core to maintain alignment and prevent leaning forward or backward.

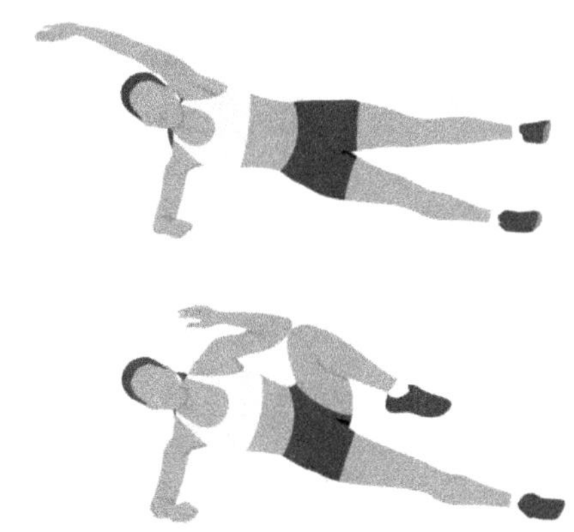

3. **Bird Dog with Tuck**
   This balancing move combines core stability with coordination, targeting the deep core muscles.
   - o **Execution**: In a tabletop position, extend one arm and the opposite leg outward. Bring your elbow and knee

o to meet in the center, engaging the core. Extend back out and repeat.
  o **Tip**: Focus on slow, controlled movements to maintain balance.

6-Minute Workout Routines

Two Advanced Routines Designed to Maximize Strength, Control, and Core Resilience

Each routine in this chapter integrates advanced moves, challenging your core stability, strength, and endurance in a quick and efficient sequence.

Routine 1: Power Core
Purpose: Builds strength and explosive power through controlled movement and holds.

- **V-Ups** (45 seconds): Focus on a smooth, controlled movement, lifting and lowering with core engagement.
- **Plank to Pike** (45 seconds): Flow between plank and pike positions, keeping your hips controlled.
- **Jackknife** (45 seconds): Lift with precision and lower slowly to maximize the burn.
- **Single-Leg Plank** (30 seconds per side): Hold a plank while lifting one leg, switching halfway through.

- **Side Plank with Leg Lift** (30 seconds per side): Keep your body in alignment as you lift and hold each leg.
- **Bicycle Crunches** (45 seconds): Slow and controlled, focusing on core engagement rather than speed.

Routine 2: Stability and Endurance Core
Purpose: Focuses on balance, control, and deep core activation for lasting core endurance.

- **Bird Dog with Tuck** (45 seconds per side): Reach and tuck slowly, keeping core stability.
- **Shoulder Tap Plank** (45 seconds): Alternate shoulder taps while keeping your hips steady.
- **Side Plank (with Optional Leg Lift)** (30 seconds per side): Hold a side plank, with or without leg lifts.
- **Single-Leg Lowering** (45 seconds): Lie on your back, lower one leg at a time, engaging the lower core.
- **Russian Twist** (45 seconds): Twist slowly, focusing on oblique activation.
- **Mountain Climbers (Slow)** (45 seconds): Perform slow, deliberate climbers to finish strong.

Final Tips for Success in Advanced Core Training

1. **Focus on Quality over Quantity**
Prioritize slow, controlled movements to maximize muscle engagement. These exercises require balance and precision, so aim to maintain form throughout each set.
2. **Listen to Your Body**
Advanced moves challenge the core but should not cause discomfort in the lower back or neck. Engage the deep core and adjust as needed, especially if you feel strain.
3. **Stay Consistent**
Regular practice of these advanced routines will yield greater strength, control, and resilience. Stick to a schedule to ensure progress without overloading the muscles.

Week 5: Cardio Core Blasts – Burn Fat While Toning

Goal: Add cardio elements to your workout to enhance calorie burn, improve endurance, and tone your core muscles for maximum results.

Cardio-core integration is a game-changer for anyone looking to elevate their fitness. This week focuses on combining core-strengthening exercises with bursts of cardiovascular activity to achieve a balanced, high-intensity workout. By engaging both your cardiovascular and muscular systems simultaneously, you'll torch calories while building a strong, stable core.

Chapter 9: Combining Core and Cardio for Maximum Results

The Benefits of Cardio-Core Integration

1. **Enhanced Fat Burning:**
   When cardio and core exercises are combined, your heart rate remains elevated throughout the workout. This sustained effort increases your caloric expenditure and optimizes fat-burning potential, especially when paired with a well-balanced diet.
2. **Improved Endurance and Stamina:**
   Cardio bursts, such as high knees or

mountain climbers, challenge your cardiovascular system, enhancing your aerobic capacity. Over time, this builds endurance, allowing you to perform more demanding exercises with less fatigue.

3. **Strengthened Core Stability:** While traditional cardio workouts often neglect the core, integrating core-focused movements such as plank jacks or Russian twists ensures you develop strength in your abdominal muscles, obliques, and lower back. A strong core improves posture, balance, and overall athletic performance.

4. **Efficiency and Time-Saving:** Combining cardio and core exercises allows you to work multiple muscle groups simultaneously, making your workouts more efficient. This approach is perfect for individuals with limited time who want to maximize results in a shorter session.

5. **Versatility:** Cardio-core workouts can be adapted for various fitness levels by modifying the intensity, duration, or complexity of exercises. This makes them ideal for beginners and advanced athletes alike.

Guidelines for Safe Cardio Integration

To get the most out of your cardio-core workouts, it's crucial to prioritize safety and maintain proper form throughout each movement.

1. **Warm-Up Thoroughly:**
   Before diving into cardio-core exercises,
   spend at least 5–10 minutes warming up.
   Incorporate dynamic stretches, light
   jogging, or movements that mimic the
   upcoming exercises, such as arm circles and
   standing twists.
2. **Focus on Form:**
   o Ensure that your core is engaged
     during every movement. For
     example, keep your abs tight and
     your spine neutral during planks or
     mountain climbers.
   o Avoid letting your lower back sag or
     arch excessively, as this can lead to
     strain and injury.
3. **Start Slowly:**
   If you're new to combining cardio and core,
   begin with lower-intensity exercises like
   standing marches paired with knee drives.
   Gradually increase intensity as you build
   confidence and endurance.
4. **Monitor Your Breathing:**
   Controlled breathing is essential during
   high-intensity intervals. Exhale during
   exertion (e.g., when pulling your knees
   toward your chest in a plank) and inhale
   during the release.
5. **Use Proper Footwear and
   Equipment:**
   o Wear supportive shoes with good
     cushioning to reduce the impact on
     your joints during cardio bursts.

- o Use a non-slip exercise mat for core-focused movements like planks and sit-ups.

6. **Incorporate Active Recovery:**
Transition from high-intensity cardio bursts to lower-intensity core movements to give your body time to recover without fully resting. This approach maintains your heart rate and maximizes calorie burn.

7. **Listen to Your Body:**
If you experience discomfort or fatigue, pause and adjust your movements. Overexertion can lead to poor form, increasing the risk of injury.

8. **Cool Down and Stretch:**
After completing your workout, spend 5–10 minutes cooling down. Include stretches that target your core and lower body, such as cobra pose and seated forward folds, to enhance flexibility and promote recovery.

Sample Cardio-Core Workout Routine (30 Minutes)

1. **Warm-Up (5 Minutes):**
   - o Jumping jacks (1 minute)
   - o Torso twists (1 minute)
   - o High knees with arm swings (1 minute)
   - o Dynamic side lunges (1 minute)
   - o Arm circles and deep breathing (1 minute)

2. **Workout Circuit (20 Minutes):** Repeat the following circuit 3 times with 1-minute rest between rounds:
   - **Plank Jacks (40 seconds):** Maintain a plank position and jump your feet apart and together.
   - **Russian Twists with Medicine Ball (40 seconds):** Sit on the floor, lean back slightly, and twist side to side with a weight or ball.
   - **High Knees (40 seconds):** Jog in place, lifting your knees as high as possible.
   - **Bicycle Crunches (40 seconds):** Alternate bringing opposite elbow and knee together while lying on your back.
   - **Mountain Climbers (40 seconds):** From a plank position, drive your knees toward your chest alternately at a quick pace.
3. **Cool Down (5 Minutes):**
   - Cat-cow stretch (1 minute)
   - Cobra pose (1 minute)
   - Child's pose (1 minute)
   - Standing forward fold (1 minute)
   - Deep breathing with side stretches (1 minute)

Chapter 10: High-Intensity Core Workouts

Ready to take your core training to the next level? This chapter focuses on high-intensity exercises that combine cardio elements with core engagement to maximize fat burning and build strength. These routines are fast-paced, efficient, and designed to push your limits while sculpting a powerful core.

Exercises with Cardio Components

High-intensity core exercises aren't just about strength; they get your heart pumping for an added calorie-burning effect. Here are three dynamic moves that combine cardio bursts with core activation:

1. **Burpees with Core Focus**
   - **How to Do It:** Start in a standing position. Drop into a squat and place your hands on the ground. Jump your feet back into a plank position, perform a push-up (optional), then jump your feet back to your hands. Explode upward into a jump and repeat.
   - **Core Engagement Tip:** Keep your core tight throughout the movement to protect your lower back and enhance abdominal activation.

- **Benefits:** Full-body conditioning, cardio endurance, and core stabilization.

2. **Plank Jacks**
   - **How to Do It:** Begin in a high plank position, with shoulders over wrists and feet together. Jump your feet apart and together, maintaining a strong plank posture.
   - **Core Engagement Tip:** Avoid letting your hips sag; keep your pelvis neutral and abs engaged.
   - **Benefits:** Cardiovascular boost and core stability improvement.

3. **High Knees with Twist**
   - **How to Do It:** Jog in place, bringing your knees as high as possible. As your knee comes up, twist your torso slightly to touch the opposite elbow to your knee.
   - **Core Engagement Tip:** Focus on twisting through the obliques for a deeper core workout.
   - **Benefits:** Elevates heart rate, strengthens the obliques, and improves coordination.

Interval-Based Core Routines

High-intensity interval training (HIIT) is an effective way to torch calories while strengthening your core. Below are two sample routines that blend cardio and core exercises for maximum impact.

Routine 1: Core Blaster Circuit (20 Minutes)

Format: Perform each exercise for 40 seconds, followed by 20 seconds of rest. Complete 3 rounds, resting for 1 minute between rounds.

1. Burpees with Core Focus
2. Plank Jacks
3. High Knees with Twist
4. Mountain Climbers
5. Bicycle Crunches

Why It Works: This routine alternates between high-intensity cardio bursts and core-focused exercises, keeping your heart rate elevated and targeting all areas of your core.

Routine 2: Tabata Core Burn (16 Minutes)

Format: Perform 20 seconds of work followed by 10 seconds of rest. Repeat each exercise for 8 rounds before moving to the next.

1. **Plank-to-Shoulder Taps:** From a plank, alternate tapping each shoulder while maintaining a strong core.

2. **Side Plank Dips:** Lower and lift your hips while holding a side plank, alternating sides every 4 rounds.
3. **Squat-to-Knee Drive:** From a squat, stand and drive one knee toward your chest, alternating legs each round.
4. **Jackknife Sit-Ups:** Lie on your back and simultaneously lift your upper body and legs to meet in the middle.

Why It Works: Tabata intervals maximize fat burning and challenge your endurance while building core strength.

Pro Tips for High-Intensity Core Workouts

1. **Focus on Quality Over Speed:** Ensure proper form during each exercise to prevent injuries and maximize results.
2. **Modify When Needed:** Beginners can reduce the intensity by stepping instead of jumping or decreasing the duration of work intervals.
3. **Use a Timer:** Keep track of intervals with a fitness timer or app to maintain the pace and structure of your workout.
4. **Hydrate and Recover:** High-intensity exercises are demanding; drink water before and after your session, and allow for adequate rest between workouts.

By incorporating high-energy moves and interval-based routines, these workouts challenge your stamina, strengthen your core, and amplify your calorie burn. With dedication, you'll see improvements in endurance, power, and overall fitness by the end of this phase. Dive in and feel the burn!

Week 6: Maintaining Core Health and Flexibility

Goal: Strengthen and stretch your core muscles to enhance resilience, prevent injury, and promote overall well-being.

After weeks of intense training, it's vital to focus on recovery and flexibility. This week emphasizes maintaining a healthy, strong, and supple core through stretching and mobility work. Core recovery ensures you can continue building strength without risking burnout or injury.

Chapter 11: Stretching and Mobility for Core Recovery

The Importance of Recovery

1. **Muscle Repair and Growth:** Recovery time allows your core muscles to repair micro-tears caused by intense workouts. This process not only strengthens the muscles but also prevents overtraining.
2. **Improved Flexibility:** Stretching lengthens tight muscles, enhancing the range of motion in your core and surrounding areas like your hips and lower back. Increased flexibility reduces the risk of strains during future workouts.
3. **Enhanced Mobility:** Mobility exercises keep the spine and torso fluid and functional, which is essential for performing everyday movements and advanced fitness routines.
4. **Stress Relief:** Core stretches and gentle mobility work promote relaxation, helping to release physical and mental tension accumulated during training.
5. **Injury Prevention:** Neglecting recovery can lead to tightness and imbalances, increasing the risk of injury. Regular stretching and mobility work maintain balance and symmetry in the core.

Key Stretches for Core Flexibility

Incorporate these stretches at the end of your workout or as part of a dedicated recovery session.

1. **Cobra Stretch (Spinal Extension)**
   - **How to Do It:** Lie face down on a mat. Place your hands under your shoulders and slowly press up, extending your spine while keeping your hips on the ground.
   - **Focus:** Stretching the abdominals and opening the chest.
   - **Benefits:** Alleviates lower back tension and promotes spinal flexibility.
2. **Seated Twist (Spinal Rotation)**
   - **How to Do It:** Sit with both legs extended forward. Cross one leg over the other, placing the foot flat on the ground. Rotate your torso toward the bent leg, placing your opposite elbow outside the knee for leverage.
   - **Focus:** Stretching the obliques and spinal muscles.
   - **Benefits:** Improves rotational flexibility and relieves tension in the lower back and sides.
3. **Child's Pose (Spinal Flexion)**
   - **How to Do It:** Sit back on your heels and stretch your arms forward

on the mat, lowering your chest toward the ground. Let your forehead rest on the mat and breathe deeply.
- o **Focus:** Stretching the lower back, abdominals, and shoulders.
- o **Benefits:** Promotes relaxation, relieves tension in the back, and lengthens the spine.

4. **Cat-Cow Stretch (Dynamic Spinal Mobility)**
   - o **How to Do It:** Start on all fours. Alternate between arching your back upward (cat pose) and lowering your belly toward the mat while lifting your head and tailbone (cow pose).
   - o **Focus:** Dynamic movement through the spine.
   - o **Benefits:** Improves mobility and relieves stiffness in the entire core and back.

5. **Side Stretch (Lateral Flexion)**
   - o **How to Do It:** Stand or sit with your arms overhead. Lean to one side, feeling a stretch along your opposite oblique and side body. Alternate sides.
   - o **Focus:** Stretching the sides and obliques.
   - o **Benefits:** Increases lateral flexibility and counteracts stiffness from sitting or repetitive motions.

Sample Core Recovery Routine (15 Minutes)

Warm-Up (3 Minutes):

- Gentle torso twists and deep breathing to prepare your body for stretching.

Main Stretches (10 Minutes):

1. Cobra Stretch (1 minute)
2. Seated Twist (1 minute per side)
3. Child's Pose (2 minutes)
4. Cat-Cow Stretch (1 minute)
5. Side Stretch (1 minute per side)

Cool Down (2 Minutes):

- Lie flat in a supine position, practicing deep diaphragmatic breathing. Focus on relaxing your core and releasing any residual tension.

By dedicating time to recovery and flexibility, you're not just soothing sore muscles—you're laying the groundwork for sustained strength and mobility. These stretches will help keep your core healthy, functional, and ready for whatever challenges come next. Embrace this restorative phase and enjoy the benefits of a resilient core!

Chapter 12: Core Mobility and Flexibility Routines

Flexibility and mobility are often overlooked but are essential components of a strong, healthy core. This chapter introduces a targeted stretching routine for flexibility and recovery, followed by insights into how combining mobility with strength can optimize your fitness results.

Core Stretching Routine: A Gentle, 6-Minute Sequence

This 6-minute stretching routine is designed to improve flexibility, relieve tension, and support core recovery. Perform it at the end of your workout or as a standalone session on rest days.

1. Cat-Cow Stretch (1 Minute)

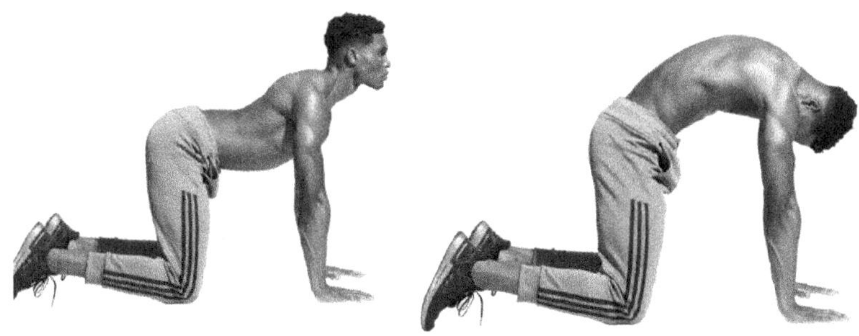

- **How to Do It:** Begin on all fours. Alternate between arching your back upward (cat pose) and lowering your belly while lifting your head and tailbone (cow pose).
- **Focus:** Mobilizing the spine and gently stretching the abdominals and back.
- **Breathing:** Inhale as you drop into cow pose and exhale as you rise into cat pose.

2. Seated Side Stretch (1 Minute)

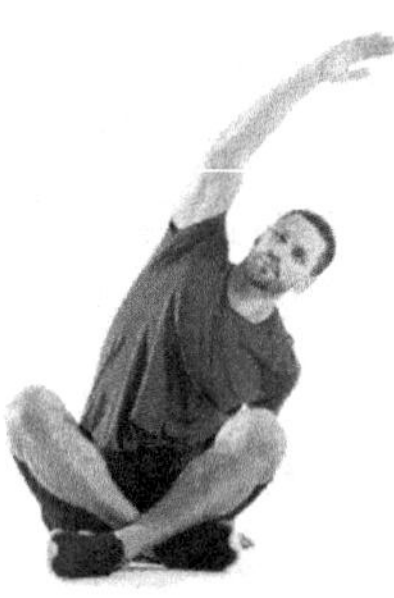

- **How to Do It:** Sit cross-legged or with legs extended. Reach one arm overhead and lean to the opposite side, stretching the obliques. Switch sides after 30 seconds.
- **Focus:** Stretching the sides of your torso and increasing lateral flexibility.
- **Tip:** Keep your sitting bones grounded to maximize the stretch.

3. Cobra Pose (1 Minute)

- **How to Do It:** Lie face down on the mat. Place your hands beneath your shoulders and press upward, extending your spine.
- **Focus:** Opening the chest and stretching the abdominals.
- **Modification:** Keep elbows slightly bent if the full extension is too intense.

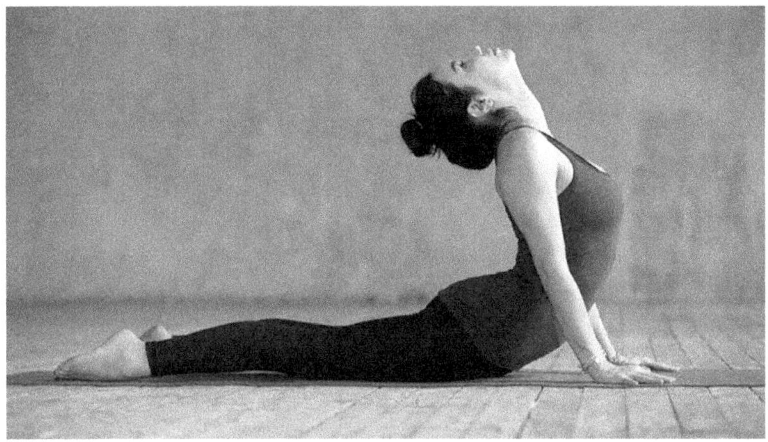

5. Spinal Twist (1 Minute)

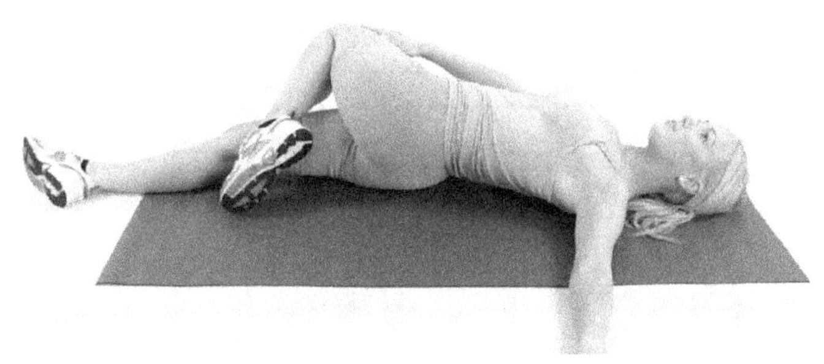

- **How to Do It:** Lie on your back, bend your knees, and drop them to one side while keeping your shoulders flat on the ground. Hold for 30 seconds, then switch sides.
- **Focus:** Releasing tension in the lower back and stretching the obliques.

6. Child's Pose (1 Minute)

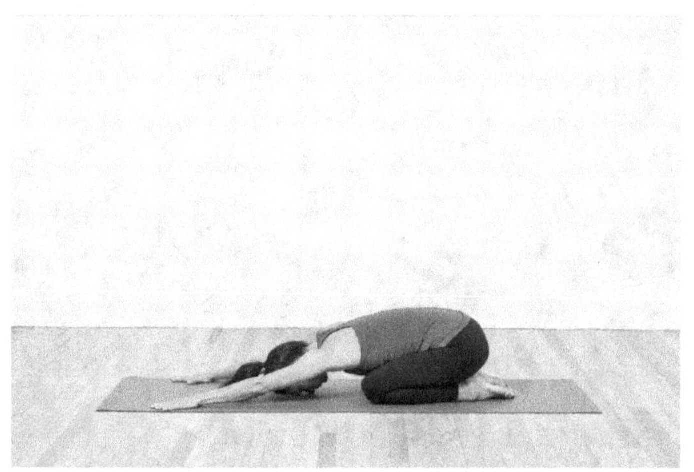

- **How to Do It:** Sit back on your heels, stretching your arms forward on the mat. Lower your chest and forehead toward the ground.
- **Focus:** Stretching the lower back and relieving tension in the hips.
- **Breathing:** Take slow, deep breaths to maximize relaxation.

6. Supine Stretch (1 Minute)

- **How to Do It:** Lie on your back with arms overhead and legs extended. Reach your arms and legs in opposite directions, creating a full-body stretch.
- **Focus:** Lengthening the spine and relaxing the entire core.
- **Tip:** Flex your feet to enhance the stretch along the lower back and hamstrings.

Combining Strength and Flexibility: The Power of Mobility

Strength and flexibility go hand in hand. Incorporating mobility exercises into your routine not only enhances recovery but also improves strength training outcomes.

Benefits of Mobility and Flexibility in Core Training

1. **Improved Range of Motion:** Flexible muscles and mobile joints allow for deeper, more effective movements in strength exercises like planks and Russian twists.
2. **Reduced Risk of Injury:** Mobility work helps prevent overuse injuries by maintaining balance and stability in the core and surrounding muscles.
3. **Enhanced Strength Gains:** A flexible core allows for better engagement

of muscles during strength training, leading to improved power and endurance.

4. **Better Posture and Alignment:** Mobility exercises support proper spinal alignment, reducing strain on the lower back and improving overall posture.

How to Combine Strength and Flexibility

1. **Dynamic Warm-Ups:** Begin your workouts with mobility-focused movements such as Cat-Cow stretches or torso twists to prepare your core for strength exercises.
2. **Active Recovery Days:** Dedicate one or two sessions per week to mobility and flexibility work to complement your strength training regimen.
3. **Integrated Movements:** Combine strength and flexibility within a single exercise. For example:
   - **Plank-to-Downward Dog:** Strengthens the core while stretching the hamstrings and shoulders.
   - **Side Plank with Hip Dips:** Engages the obliques while improving lateral mobility.
4. **Cool-Down Routines:** End each workout with static stretches from the 6-minute routine to relax the muscles and improve flexibility over time.

By balancing strength with flexibility and mobility, you create a foundation for long-term core health and performance. This chapter empowers you with tools to stretch, recover, and train smarter, ensuring your core remains both strong and resilient.

Chapter 13: Nutrition for a Lean, Strong Core

Building a lean, strong core isn't just about exercise—it's also about what you put on your plate. Proper nutrition fuels your workouts, supports muscle recovery, and helps reveal the toned core you're working hard to achieve. This chapter focuses on the critical role of diet in core definition, highlights foods that promote muscle health and reduce bloating, and provides sample meal plans to make eating for a lean core simple and sustainable.

The Role of Diet in Core Definition

1. **Balancing Caloric Intake:**
   - To achieve a lean core, you need to manage your calorie intake. A moderate calorie deficit helps burn fat while preserving muscle mass, revealing the definition in your core muscles.
2. **Prioritizing Protein:**
   - Protein is vital for muscle repair and growth, especially after core-intensive workouts. Aim for lean protein sources such as chicken, fish, eggs, tofu, and legumes.
3. **Controlling Carbohydrates:**

- While carbs provide energy, focus on complex carbohydrates like quinoa, brown rice, and sweet potatoes to avoid blood sugar spikes and crashes.
4. **Healthy Fats for Hormonal Balance:**
   - Incorporate healthy fats like avocados, nuts, seeds, and olive oil. These fats support hormone regulation, which is crucial for fat metabolism.
5. **Hydration Matters:**
   - Staying hydrated reduces bloating, improves digestion, and helps maintain energy levels for your workouts.

Core-Friendly Foods

Incorporate these foods into your diet to support muscle health, reduce bloating, and promote a leaner core:

Nutrients for Core Strength:

- **Protein:** Chicken breast, salmon, eggs, Greek yogurt, tofu.
- **Fiber:** Leafy greens, broccoli, berries, oats.
- **Healthy Fats:** Avocados, almonds, chia seeds, walnuts.
- **Complex Carbohydrates:** Quinoa, sweet potatoes, brown rice.

Foods to Reduce Bloating:

- **Ginger:** Soothes digestion and reduces bloating.
- **Peppermint Tea:** Calms the digestive system.
- **Bananas:** High in potassium to counter sodium-induced bloating.
- **Cucumber and Celery:** Natural diuretics that help flush excess water.

Sample Meal Plans and Tips

Here's a sample day of meals designed to fuel your workouts, reduce bloating, and support a lean, strong core.

Breakfast

Avocado and Egg Toast:

- 1 slice of whole-grain bread
- ½ avocado, mashed
- 1 poached egg
- Sprinkle of red pepper flakes
- **Why it works:** High in protein, healthy fats, and fiber for sustained energy.

Optional Add-On: A cup of green tea for its metabolism-boosting properties.

Mid-Morning Snack

Greek Yogurt with Berries:

- ½ cup Greek yogurt (unsweetened)
- Handful of mixed berries (blueberries, raspberries)
- 1 teaspoon chia seeds
- **Why it works:** Packed with protein, antioxidants, and fiber.

Lunch

Quinoa and Grilled Chicken Salad:

- 1 cup cooked quinoa
- 3 oz grilled chicken breast
- Mixed greens, cherry tomatoes, cucumbers
- Dressing: Olive oil and lemon juice
- **Why it works:** Balanced with lean protein, complex carbs, and healthy fats.

Afternoon Snack

Veggie Sticks with Hummus:

- Slices of cucumber, bell peppers, and carrots
- 2 tablespoons hummus

- **Why it works:** Provides fiber and healthy fats to keep you full until dinner.

Dinner

Baked Salmon with Steamed Broccoli and Sweet Potatoes:

- 3 oz baked salmon (seasoned with garlic and dill)
- 1 cup steamed broccoli
- ½ medium sweet potato, roasted
- **Why it works:** Combines omega-3s, fiber, and complex carbs to support recovery and reduce inflammation.

Evening Option

Chamomile Tea:

- 1 cup of chamomile tea before bed to relax and support digestion.

Tips for Long-Term Success

1. **Meal Prep:**
   Plan and prepare meals in advance to make

healthy eating convenient. Use containers for portion control.

2. **Mindful Eating:**
Eat slowly and pay attention to your body's hunger and fullness cues. This practice helps prevent overeating and supports digestion.

3. **Balance, Not Deprivation:**
Enjoy your favorite foods occasionally in moderation. Balance is key to sustainability.

4. **Track Your Progress:**
Keep a food journal or use apps to monitor your nutrition and ensure you're meeting your goals.

By combining smart nutrition with your workout plan, you'll fuel your body effectively and reveal the lean, strong core you've worked hard to build. This approach not only enhances your physical appearance but also supports overall health and well-being.

Chapter 14: Creating a Sustainable Core Routine

A strong, healthy core is a lifelong asset, but maintaining it requires consistency and adaptability. In this chapter, we explore how to establish long-term habits, adapt workouts as your fitness evolves, and structure flexible weekly core schedules to fit your lifestyle and goals.

Establishing Long-Term Habits

Consistency is the cornerstone of fitness success. To keep core training a regular part of your routine, consider the following strategies:

1. **Set Realistic Goals:**
   - Define what you want to achieve, whether it's improved posture, enhanced athletic performance, or visible muscle definition.
   - Break larger goals into smaller milestones to keep motivation high.
2. **Make Core Training a Priority:**
   - Schedule specific times for core workouts, treating them as non-negotiable appointments.
   - Incorporate core exercises into your existing workout routine (e.g., adding planks to a cardio day).
3. **Track Your Progress:**

- o Use a fitness journal or app to log your workouts, noting improvements in strength, endurance, or form.
  - o Celebrate small wins, like holding a plank for an extra 10 seconds or mastering a challenging exercise.
4. **Stay Engaged:**
  - o Vary your workouts to prevent boredom. Alternate between static exercises like planks and dynamic moves like Russian twists or mountain climbers.
  - o Experiment with new tools such as stability balls, resistance bands, or Pilates-inspired routines.

Adapting Workouts to Your Progress

Your fitness needs and abilities will evolve over time. Here's how to keep your core routine effective and aligned with your progress:

1. **Increase Intensity Gradually:**
  - o Add weight to core exercises like weighted sit-ups or Russian twists.
  - o Increase the duration or repetitions of bodyweight exercises (e.g., extend plank holds or do more flutter kicks).
2. **Modify for Challenges:**
  - o If an exercise feels too easy, introduce variations. For instance,

progress from standard planks to side planks or plank jacks.
   - Incorporate compound movements, such as combining squats with core twists.
3. **Address Plateaus:**
   - If progress stalls, mix things up with new exercises, HIIT-based core sessions, or yoga-inspired stretches to re-engage the muscles.
4. **Adjust for Life Changes:**
   - During busy periods, focus on shorter, high-impact workouts like a 10-minute core blast.
   - For recovery phases or lower energy days, prioritize stretching and mobility routines.

Sample Weekly Core Schedules

Below are flexible schedules tailored to different fitness levels, time availability, and goals.

Option 1: Beginner Schedule (3 Days Per Week)

Goal: Build foundational strength and consistency.

- **Monday:** Core Basics

o   3 rounds of 30-second planks, 15 leg raises, and 20 Russian twists.
- **Wednesday:** Stability Focus
  o   3 rounds of 15 bird-dogs, 10 seated twists, and 20 glute bridges.
- **Friday:** Core Mobility
  o   6-minute stretching routine (Child's Pose, Cobra, Cat-Cow).

Option 2: Intermediate Schedule (4 Days Per Week)

Goal: Enhance strength and endurance with moderate intensity.

- **Monday:** Strength Core
  o   3 rounds of 30-second side planks (each side), 20 flutter kicks, and 15 weighted sit-ups.
- **Tuesday:** Recovery and Flexibility
  o   Core-focused yoga flow (Cobra, Spinal Twist, Seated Side Stretch).
- **Thursday:** Cardio Core
  o   20-minute interval routine alternating 1 minute of high knees with 1 minute of plank jacks.
- **Saturday:** Total Core Burn
  o   3 rounds of 20 mountain climbers, 15 V-ups, and 10 hanging leg raises.

Option 3: Advanced Schedule (5 Days Per Week)

Goal: Maintain a highly developed core with variety and intensity.

- **Monday:** Weighted Core
    - 3 rounds of 20 weighted Russian twists, 15 hanging leg raises, and 10 ab rollouts.
- **Wednesday:** Core Cardio Blast
    - 25-minute HIIT workout alternating 30 seconds of burpees with 1 minute of bicycle crunches.
- **Friday:** Core Endurance
    - 2-minute plank holds, 3 rounds of 20 mountain climbers, and 15 jackknife sit-ups.
- **Saturday:** Recovery Stretch
    - 10-minute yoga sequence focusing on spinal twists, Child's Pose, and Cobra stretches.
- **Sunday:** Functional Core
    - Compound movements like kettlebell swings, medicine ball slams, or woodchoppers.

Tips for Maintaining a Sustainable Routine

1. **Listen to Your Body:**
    - Rest if you feel fatigued or sore. Core recovery is just as crucial as training.

2. **Keep It Fun:**
   - o   Invite friends or family to join your workouts for added motivation.
3. **Stay Inspired:**
   - o   Follow fitness influencers, join online classes, or track your progress visually with before-and-after photos.

By making core workouts a consistent and adaptable part of your fitness routine, you'll enjoy the benefits of a strong, resilient core for years to come.

Chapter 15: Measuring Progress and Staying Motivated

Tracking your journey and staying motivated are essential for long-term success in core training. This chapter focuses on how to measure your physical changes effectively, maintain your drive, and celebrate milestones to keep you committed to your fitness goals.

Tracking Physical Changes

Monitoring your progress is crucial for understanding what's working and where you need to improve. Here's how to track your gains in strength, endurance, and aesthetics:

1. **Strength Progress:**
   - **Core Exercises:** Note the number of repetitions or the duration of exercises like planks, sit-ups, or leg raises. For example, if you increase your plank hold from 30 seconds to 90 seconds, that's measurable progress.
   - **Weight Progression:** Track how much weight you can add to core-strengthening exercises like Russian twists or weighted sit-ups.
2. **Endurance Gains:**
   - **Workout Duration:** Measure how long you can maintain a high-

intensity core workout without needing rest.

- o **Recovery Time:** Track how quickly you recover from a challenging routine—shorter recovery times indicate improved endurance.

3. **Aesthetic Changes:**
   - o **Body Composition:** Use a tape measure to monitor changes in your waistline, hips, and abdominal region.
   - o **Photos:** Take progress pictures at regular intervals (e.g., every two weeks) to visually track improvements in core definition.
   - o **Body Fat Percentage:** If available, use tools like body fat scales or professional assessments to measure changes.

Maintaining Motivation

Staying motivated is key to sustaining your core routine, especially during plateaus or busy times. Use these strategies to keep moving forward:

1. **Set Achievable Goals:**
   - o Break larger fitness goals into smaller, manageable milestones. For instance, aim to improve your plank time by 15 seconds each week.

- o Focus on performance-based goals, such as mastering a challenging move like a hanging leg raise or progressing to advanced side planks.
2. **Track and Reflect:**
   - o Keep a fitness journal or use an app to log your workouts, diet, and progress.
   - o Review your entries regularly to recognize patterns, successes, and areas for improvement.
3. **Find Your Why:**
   - o Reflect on why you started your core journey—whether it's to improve posture, reduce back pain, or feel confident in your body.
   - o Use this purpose as a source of inspiration during challenging moments.
4. **Combat Plateaus:**
   - o Vary your workouts by adding new exercises, increasing intensity, or switching to a different training style (e.g., yoga-based core flows).
   - o Reward yourself for sticking with the routine—treat yourself to new workout gear or a relaxing massage.

Celebrating Successes

Recognizing your achievements, big or small, keeps your mindset positive and reinforces your commitment.

1. **Celebrate Milestones:**
   - Honor personal bests, such as holding a plank for two minutes or completing a high-intensity interval workout without breaks.
   - Reward non-aesthetic milestones like reduced back pain, improved posture, or increased daily energy.
2. **Share Your Wins:**
   - Tell a friend, family member, or fitness community about your progress to amplify your sense of accomplishment.
   - Social accountability and encouragement from others can boost motivation.
3. **Focus on Progress, Not Perfection:**
   - Understand that fitness is a journey, not a destination. Even small improvements, like mastering better form, are worth celebrating.

Practical Tools for Measuring and Staying Motivated

- **Tracking Apps:** Use fitness apps like MyFitnessPal or Strava to monitor your activity and achievements.

- **Wearables:** Fitness trackers can measure your activity, heart rate, and calorie burn.
- **Accountability Partners:** Partner with a workout buddy or coach who can provide support and encouragement.
- **Vision Boards:** Create a visual reminder of your goals with photos, motivational quotes, and milestones to achieve.

By measuring progress consistently, staying motivated with achievable goals, and celebrating your successes, you'll build a sustainable core routine that delivers results while keeping you inspired. Let every step forward—no matter how small—remind you of your strength and commitment to a healthier, more resilient core.

Conclusion: Embracing the Journey of Core Transformation

As we reach the final stretch of your core transformation journey, it's essential to reflect on everything you've achieved and look forward to the lasting benefits this journey brings. Building a strong, toned core isn't just about aesthetics; it's about creating a foundation for lifelong fitness, resilience, and well-being.

Final Thoughts on Core Transformation

A strong core is at the heart of your overall fitness and functional health. Here's why your efforts matter:

1. **Enhanced Physical Performance:**
   - Your core powers almost every movement, from lifting groceries to running marathons. A strong, stable core enhances balance, coordination, and agility in both workouts and daily life.
2. **Injury Prevention:**
   - By strengthening the muscles that stabilize your spine and pelvis, you've reduced the risk of common injuries, such as lower back pain or strains.
3. **Improved Posture and Confidence:**

- A well-toned core supports better posture, helping you stand taller and move with grace. This confidence radiates into other areas of your life.

4. **Functional Fitness:**
   - Your core training isn't confined to the gym—it translates into real-world strength. Whether you're playing with your kids, tackling a home project, or simply enjoying a pain-free day, your core supports it all.

5. **Mental Resilience:**
   - Beyond the physical, you've cultivated discipline, focus, and a sense of accomplishment. These mental gains are just as transformative as the physical ones.

Encouragement to Keep Moving Forward

While this program may conclude here, your core journey is far from over. Here are some parting thoughts to inspire you to continue:

1. **Consistency is Key:**
   - Remember that long-term results come from consistent effort. Even short core workouts a few times a week can maintain and build on your progress.

2. **Patience Pays Off:**

o   Fitness is a lifelong journey, not a race. Celebrate small victories along the way, and don't be discouraged by setbacks—they're a natural part of growth.

3. **Keep Challenging Yourself:**
   o   As your fitness improves, look for ways to push your limits. Try advanced core exercises, explore new fitness modalities, or set new personal goals to stay engaged and motivated.

4. **Embrace the Lifelong Benefits:**
   o   A strong core supports you at every stage of life. It helps you age gracefully, stay active, and enjoy a higher quality of life well into the future.

5. **Stay Inspired:**
   o   Surround yourself with people and resources that motivate you. Share your journey, connect with like-minded individuals, and remind yourself of why you started.

Celebrate Your Transformation

This isn't just the end of a program—it's the beginning of a new chapter in your fitness journey. You've gained more than a stronger core; you've built habits, resilience, and confidence that will serve you for years to come.

As you move forward, let the lessons from this journey inspire your next steps. Whether it's improving your strength, maintaining your flexibility, or simply living pain-free, the foundation you've built will support every goal you set.

Remember, the journey is yours to own and shape. Keep moving, stay consistent, and celebrate every success—big or small. Your core transformation is a testament to your commitment, and the best is yet to come.

Here's to your continued strength, health, and happiness!

Appendix: Tools for Your Core Journey

This appendix provides quick and practical tools to help you make the most of your core training. With a reference guide to exercises and a customizable workout calendar, you'll have everything you need to stay organized, track progress, and keep moving forward.

Quick Reference Guide to Exercises

Here's a directory of all the exercises featured in this book, along with brief instructions and common modifications to suit your fitness level.

Core Strengthening Exercises:

1. **Plank Variations:**
   - **Standard Plank:** Support yourself on forearms and toes, keeping your body in a straight line.
   - **Modification:** Drop to your knees for less intensity.
2. **Russian Twists:**
   - Sit on the floor, lean back slightly, and twist your torso side to side, tapping the floor beside you.
   - **Modification:** Keep feet on the floor or use a light weight for added resistance.
3. **Bicycle Crunches:**
   - Lie on your back, bring opposite elbow to knee in a pedaling motion.
   - **Modification:** Slow the pace to focus on form.
4. **Side Plank:**
   - Balance on one forearm and the side of your foot, keeping your body aligned.
   - **Modification:** Lower your bottom knee to the ground for added support.

Core and Cardio Combination Exercises:

1. **Burpees:**
   - Begin standing, drop into a squat, kick feet back into a plank, then return to standing with a jump.

- o **Modification:** Remove the jump for a lower-impact option.

2. **Plank Jacks:**
   - o In a plank position, jump feet apart and back together like a jumping jack.
   - o **Modification:** Step feet in and out instead of jumping.

3. **High Knees:**
   - o Run in place, bringing your knees as high as possible.
   - o **Modification:** March in place with controlled knee lifts.

Flexibility and Recovery Stretches:

1. **Cobra Pose:**
   - o Lie face down, place hands under shoulders, and lift your chest upward while keeping hips on the ground.
   - o **Modification:** Keep elbows slightly bent for less intensity.

2. **Seated Twist:**
   - o Sit with one leg extended, place the opposite foot across the extended leg, and twist toward the bent knee.
   - o **Modification:** Keep the twist gentle to avoid overstretching.

3. **Child's Pose:**
   - o Kneel on the floor, extend your arms forward, and rest your forehead on the mat.
   - o **Modification:** Place a cushion under your hips for added support.

Core Workout Calendar

Use this customizable calendar template to track your core workouts, measure your consistency, and plan your weekly routines.

Sample Template:

Day	Workout Plan	Notes/Progress
Monday	Core Strength (e.g., Plank Variations)	Increased plank hold to 1 minute
Tuesday	Rest or Light Stretching	Felt energized post-stretch
Wednesday	Cardio-Core Combo (e.g., Burpees)	Completed 3 sets, pushed hard!
Thursday	Recovery and Flexibility (e.g., Cobra)	Lower back felt much better
Friday	High-Intensity Core (e.g., Side Planks)	Maintained form throughout
Saturday	Optional Bonus	

Day	Workout Plan	Notes/Progress
	Workout or Active Recovery	
Sunday	Rest and Reflection	

How to Use the Calendar:

- **Customizable Workouts:** Fill in the exercises based on your goals and schedule.
- **Progress Notes:** Use the notes section to record how you felt, improvements, or adjustments made.
- **Reflect Weekly:** At the end of each week, review your performance and set new targets.

By combining a detailed exercise guide with a practical tracking tool, this appendix ensures you stay organized and motivated as you work toward your core goals. Use it to reinforce your commitment and enjoy the rewards of a consistent, effective routine.